Keto Vegetarian Cookbook for Beginners

Easy to Make and Delicious Low-Carb, High-Fat Vegetarian Recipes to Lose Weight

Lidia Wong

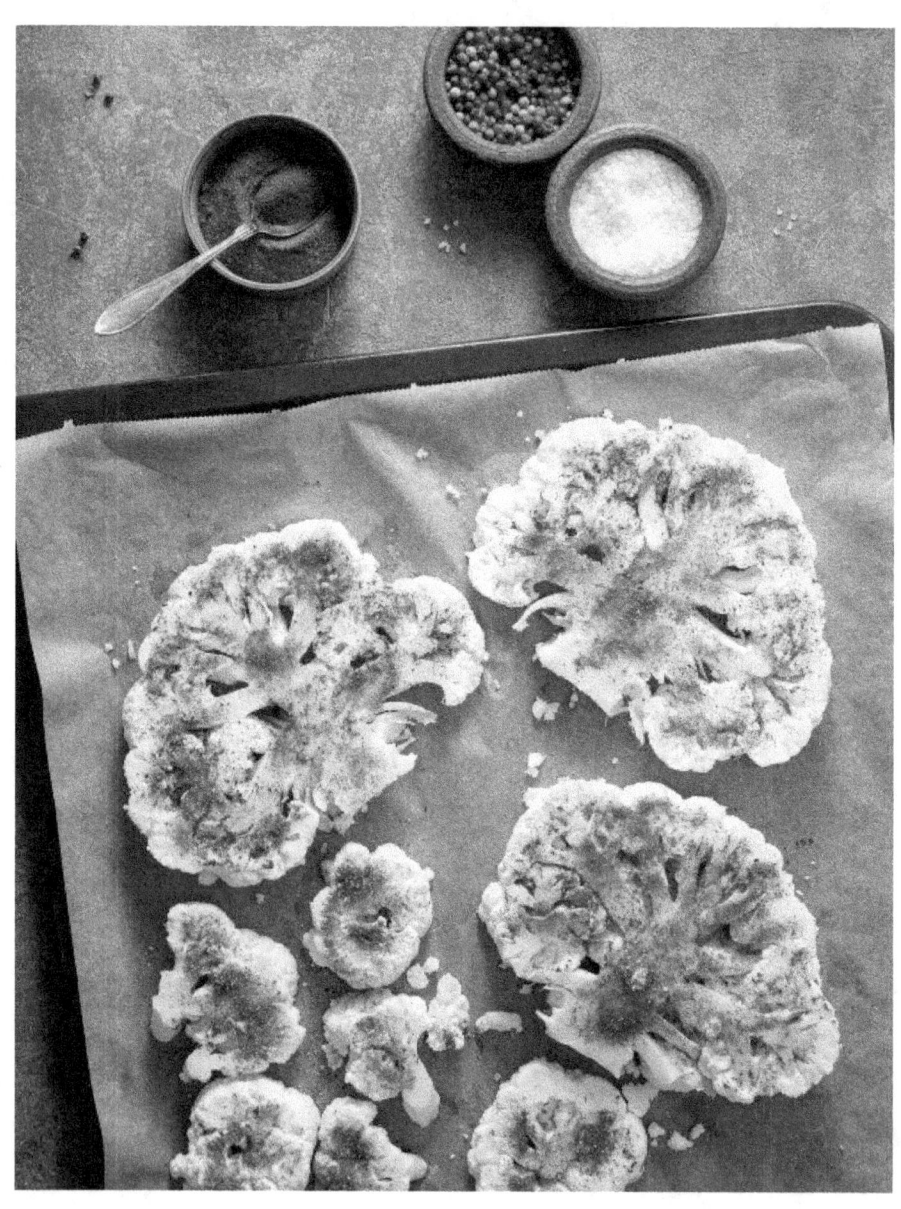

© Copyright 2021 by Lidia Wong - All rights reserved.

The content contained within this book may not be reproduced, duplicated or transmitted without direct written permission from the author or the publisher.
Under no circumstances will any blame or legal responsibility be held against the publisher, or author, for any damages, reparation, or monetary loss due to the information contained within this book. Either directly or indirectly.

Legal Notice:
This book is copyright protected. This book is only for personal use. You cannot amend, distribute, sell, use, quote or paraphrase any part, or the content within this book, without the consent of the author or publisher.

Disclaimer Notice:
Please note the information contained within this document is for educational and entertainment purposes only. All effort has been executed to present accurate, up to date, and reliable, complete information. No warranties of any kind are declared or implied. Readers acknowledge that the author is not engaging in the rendering of legal, financial, medical or professional advice. The content within this book has been derived from various sources. Please consult a licensed professional before attempting any techniques outlined in this book.
By reading this document, the reader agrees that under no circumstances is the author responsible for any losses, direct or indirect, which are incurred as a result of the use of information contained within this document, including, but not limited to, — errors, omissions, or inaccuracies.

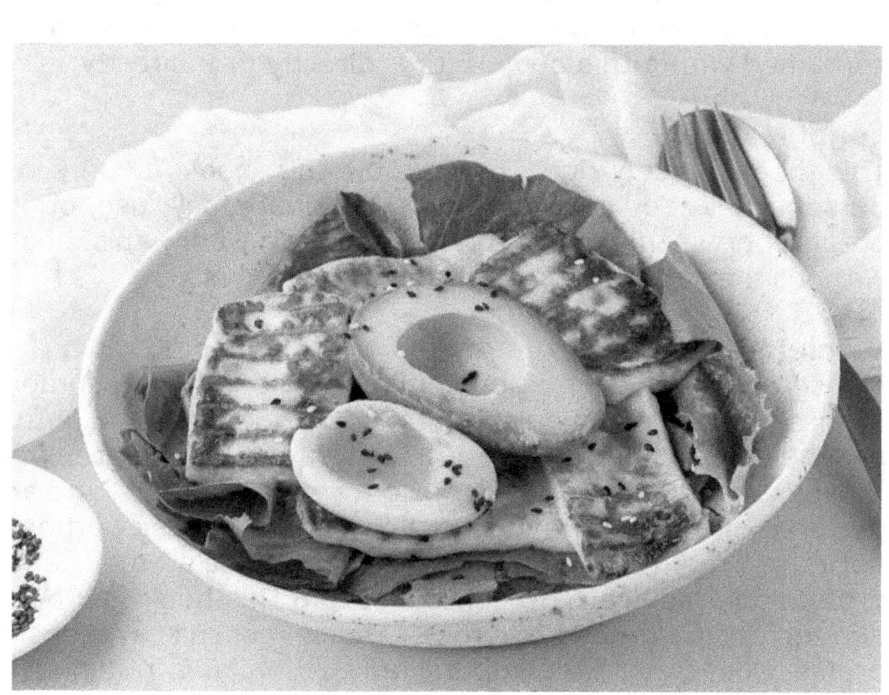

TABLE OF CONTENTS

INTRODUCTION 1

Artichoke Dip 3

Spicy Carrot Noodles 5

Creamy Zucchini Quiche 7

Vegan Sausage Collard Rolls 9

Seitan Tex-Mex Casserole 11

Tempeh with Garlic Asparagus 13

Cashew Buttered Quesadillas with Leafy Greens 15

Grapes and Tomato Salad 18

Spinach Mix 19

Balsamic Brussels Sprouts 21

Chili Asparagus 22

Sweet Potato Mash 24

Simple Potatoes Side Dish 26

Special Potatoes Mix 27

Cumin Cauliflower Rice and Broccoli 28

Radish and Broccoli 30

Mashed Broccoli 31

Roasted Cauliflower Tacos 33

Creamy Mint-Lime Spaghetti Squash ... 36

Marsala Carrots ... 39

Garlic And Herb Zoodles ... 41

Artichokes and Mushroom Mix ... 43

Orange Juice Smoothie ... 46

Vegan Rice Pudding ... 48

Asparagus Frittata ... 50

Mushroom & Wild Rice Stew ... 52

Tamarind Chickpea Stew ... 55

Pesto Parmesan Tempeh with Green Pasta ... 58

Creamy Tofu with Green Beans and Keto Fettuccine ... 60

Rice Salad With Cashews And Dried Papaya ... 63

Easy Avocado and Cremini Mushroom Melts ... 65

Potato Chips ... 67

Loaded Baked Potatoes ... 69

Almond Green Beans ... 71

Tomato Asparagus Salad ... 73

Spinach Tomato Stir Fry ... 75

Jalapeno and Cilantro Hummus ... 77

Chocolate Coconut Brownies ... 78

Avocado and Rhubarb Salad ... 81

Coconut Salad.. 82

Brown Betty Bananas Foster. 83

Smoothie Bowl... 85

Lemon Curd Dessert (Sugar Free)............................... 86

Strawberries Cream... 87

Blackberry Pie... 88

Lime Cream... 90

Quick And Easy Ranch Dip 92

Roasted Cashews 94

Brownies 95

Rich Jackfruit Dish 97

Avocado Pudding.. 99

Avocado and Almond Sweet Cream 101

NOTE **102**

INTRODUCTION

The keto diet is the shortened term for ketogenic diet and it is essentially a high-fat and low-carb diet that helps you lose weight, thereby bringing various health benefits. This diet drastically restricts your carb intake while increasing your fat intake; this pushes your body to go into a state know as "*ketosis*". We will tackle ketosis in a bit.

The human body uses glucose from carbs to fuel metabolic pathways—meaning various bodily functions like digestion, breathing, etc.. Essentially, anything that needs energy. Even when you are resting, the body needs fuel or energy for you to continue living. If you think about it, when have you ever stopped breathing, or your heart stopped beating, or your liver stopped from cleansing the body, or your kidneys from filtering blood?

Never, unless you're dead, which is the only time in which the body doesn't need energy. In normal circumstances, glucose is the primary pathway when it comes to sourcing the body's energy.

But the body also has another pathway; it can utilize fats to fuel the various bodily processes. And this is what we call "*ketosis*". And the body can only enter ketosis when there is no glucose available, thus the reason for sticking to a low-carb diet is essential in the keto diet. Since no glucose is available, the body is pushed to use fats—it can either come from the food you consume or from your body's fat reserves—the adipose tissue or from the flabby parts of your body. This is how the keto diet helps you lose weight, by burning up all those stored fats that you have and using it to fuel bodily processes.

That said, if for whatever reason you are a vegetarian, following a ketogenic diet can be extremely difficult. A vegetarian diet is largely free of animal products, which means that food tends to be usually high in carbohydrates. Still, with careful planning, it is possible. This Cookbook will provide you with various easy and delicious dishes to help you stick to your ketogenic diet plan while being a vegetarian.

Enjoy!

Artichoke Dip

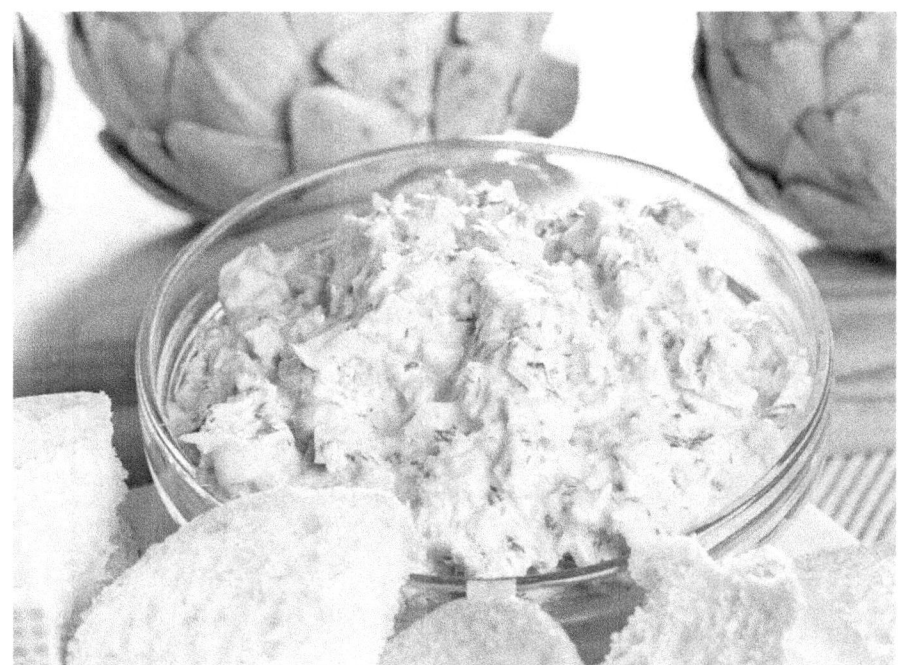

Preparation Time: 5 minutes

Cooking Time: 35 minutes

Servings: 4

Ingredients:

- 1 cup cheddar cheese, shredded
- 15-ounces artichoke hearts, drained

- 1 teaspoon Worcestershire sauce
- 3 cups arugula, chopped
- ½ cup mayonnaise
- 1 tablespoon onion, minced

Directions:

1. Preheat your oven to 350° Fahrenheit. Blend all ingredients using a blender and blend until smooth. Pour artichoke mixture into a baking dish and bake in preheated oven for 30 minutes. Serve with crackers and enjoy!

Nutritional Values (Per Serving):

Calories: 284 Fat: 19.4 g Cholesterol: 37 mg Sugar: 3.8 g Carbohydrates: 19 g Protein: 11.2 g

Spicy Carrot Noodles

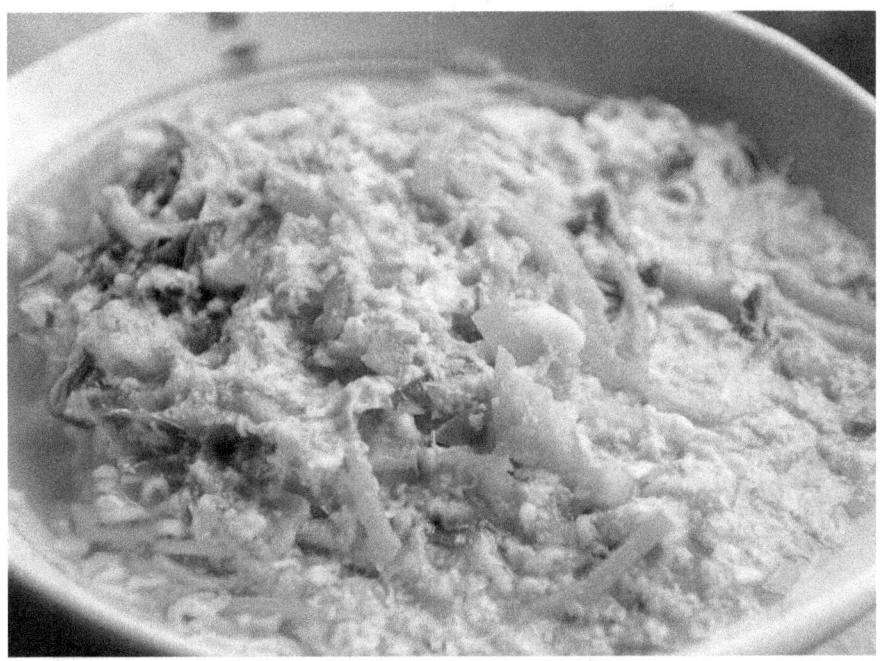

Preparation Time: 20 minutes

Servings: 3

Ingredients:

- 5 medium carrots
- 2/3 cup olive oil
- 4 tbsp red chili pepper flakes, crushed

- 1/4 cup fresh spring onions, chopped
- 1/4 cup vinegar
- 3 garlic cloves, chopped
- 1/2 cup basil leaves
- 1 cup fresh parsley
- Salt

Directions:

1. Add red chili flakes, oil, vinegar, garlic, spring onions, basil, and parsley in a blender and blend until smooth. Pour paste into a large bowl.
2. Add water in a large saucepan with little salt and bring to boil.
3. Peel carrots and using spiralizer make noodles.
4. Add carrot noodles in boiling water and blanch for 2 minutes or until softened.
5. Add cooked noodles in large bowl and toss mix well with paste.
6. Serve immediately and enjoy.

Nutritional Value (Amount per Serving):

Calories 450 Fat 45 g Carbohydrates 14 g Sugar 6 g Protein 2 g Cholesterol 0 mg

Creamy Zucchini Quiche

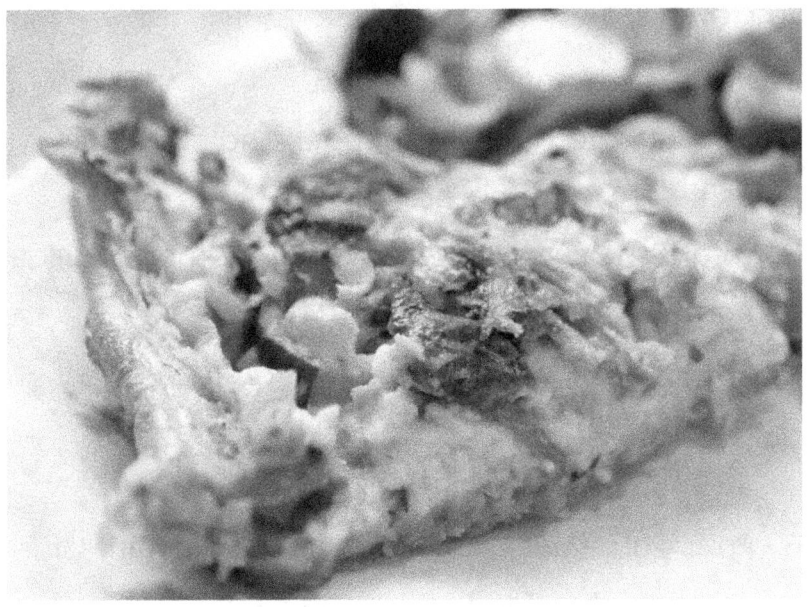

Preparation Time: 120 minutes

Servings: 8

Ingredients:

- 2 large eggs
- 2 lbs zucchini, thinly sliced
- 1 1/2 cup almond milk
- 2 cups cheddar cheese, shredded
- Pepper

- Salt

Directions:
1. Preheat the oven to 375 °F.
2. Season zucchini with pepper and salt and set aside for 30 minutes.
3. In a large bowl, beat eggs with almond milk, pepper, and salt.
4. Add shredded cheddar cheese and stir well.
5. Spray quiche pan with cooking spray and arrange zucchini slices in quiche pan.
6. Pour egg and milk mixture over zucchini the sprinkle shredded cheese.
7. Bake in preheated oven for 60 minutes or until quiche is lightly golden brown.
8. Serve warm and enjoy.

Nutritional Value (Amount per Serving):

Calories 253 Fat 21 g Carbohydrates 6 g Sugar 3 g Protein 11 g Cholesterol 76 mg

Vegan Sausage Collard Rolls

Preparation Time: 10 minutes

Cooking Time: 1 hour, 3 minutes, 30 seconds

Servings: 4

Ingredients:
- 1 lb crumbled vegan sausages
- 1 tbsp butter
- 2 tsp coconut aminos
- 1 tsp Dijon mustard
- ¼ tsp allspice
- 1 tsp whole peppercorns
- ¼ tsp cloves
- 1 medium red onion, sliced
- ½ tsp red pepper flakes
- 1 large bay leaf
- 1 lemon, zested and juiced
- ¼ cup white wine
- ¼ cup freshly brewed coffee
- 2/3 tbsp erythritol
- 8 large Swiss collard leaves
- Salt and black pepper to taste

Directions:

1. In a large pot, add all the ingredients up to the collard leaves and mix well.
2. Close the lid of the pot and cook the ingredients over low heat for 1 hour or until the vegan sausages cook.
3. 10 minutes to the time being up, boil some water in a medium pot over medium heat and add all the collards with one onion slice. Cook for 30 seconds and transfer the leaves immediately to an ice bath to blanch for 5 to 10 minutes.
4. Remove the collards, pat dry with a paper towel, and lay flat on a flat surface.
5. Divide the vegan sausages mixture onto the collards, top with the onion slices, and roll the leaves over to cover the filling.
6. Serve immediately.

Nutrition:

Calories: 356, Total Fat: 21.2g, Saturated Fat: 8.8g, Total Carbs: 10g, Dietary Fiber: 0g, Sugar: 3g, Protein:35 g, Sodium: 557mg

Seitan Tex-Mex Casserole

Preparation Time: 5 minutes

Cooking Time: 35 minutes

Serving: 4

Ingredients:

- 2 tbsp butter
- 1 ½ lb seitan
- 2 tbsp chopped jalapeño peppers
- 3 tbsp Tex-Mex seasoning
- ½ cup crushed tomatoes
- 1 tbsp chopped fresh green onion to garnish
- 1 cup sour cream for serving
- Salt and black pepper to taste
- ½ cup shredded provolone cheese

Directions:

1. Preheat the oven and grease a baking dish with cooking spray. Set aside.
2. Melt the butter in a medium skillet over medium heat and cook the seitan until brown, 10 minutes.

3. Stir in the Tex-Mex seasoning, jalapeño peppers, and tomatoes; simmer for 5 minutes and adjust the taste with salt and black pepper.
4. Transfer and level the mixture in the baking dish. Top with the provolone cheese and bake in the oven's upper rack for 15 to 20 minutes or until the cheese melts and is golden brown.
5. Remove the dish and garnish with the green onion.
6. Serve the casserole with sour cream.

Nutrition:

Calories: 464, Total Fat:37.8 g, Saturated Fat:7.4 g, Total Carbs: 12 g, Dietary Fiber: 2g, Sugar: 3g, Protein:24 g, Sodium: 147mg

Tempeh with Garlic Asparagus

Preparation Time: 10 minutes

Cooking Time: 18 minutes

Serving: 4

Ingredients:

For the tempeh:

- 4 tempeh slices
- 3 tbsp butter
- Salt and black pepper to taste

For the garlic buttered asparagus:

- 1 lb asparagus, trimmed and halved
- 2 tbsp. olive oil
- 2 garlic cloves, minced
- Salt and black pepper to taste
- 1 tbsp dried parsley
- 1 small lemon, juiced

Directions:

For the tempeh:

1. Melt the butter in a medium skillet over medium heat, season the tempeh with salt, black pepper

and fry in the butter on both sides until brown and cooked through, 10 minutes. Transfer to a plate and set aside in a warmer for serving.

For the garlic asparagus:

2. Heat the olive oil in a medium skillet over medium heat, and sauté the garlic until fragrant, 30 seconds.
3. Stir in the asparagus, season with salt and black pepper, and cook until slightly softened with a bit of crunch, 5 minutes.
4. Mix in the parsley, lemon juice, toss to coat well and plate the asparagus.
5. Serve the asparagus warm with the tempeh.

Nutrition:

Calories: 181, Total Fat:17.5 g, Saturated Fat:11 g, Total Carbs: 6 g, Dietary Fiber: 3g, Sugar: 2g, Protein: 3g, Sodium: 140mg

Cashew Buttered Quesadillas with Leafy Greens

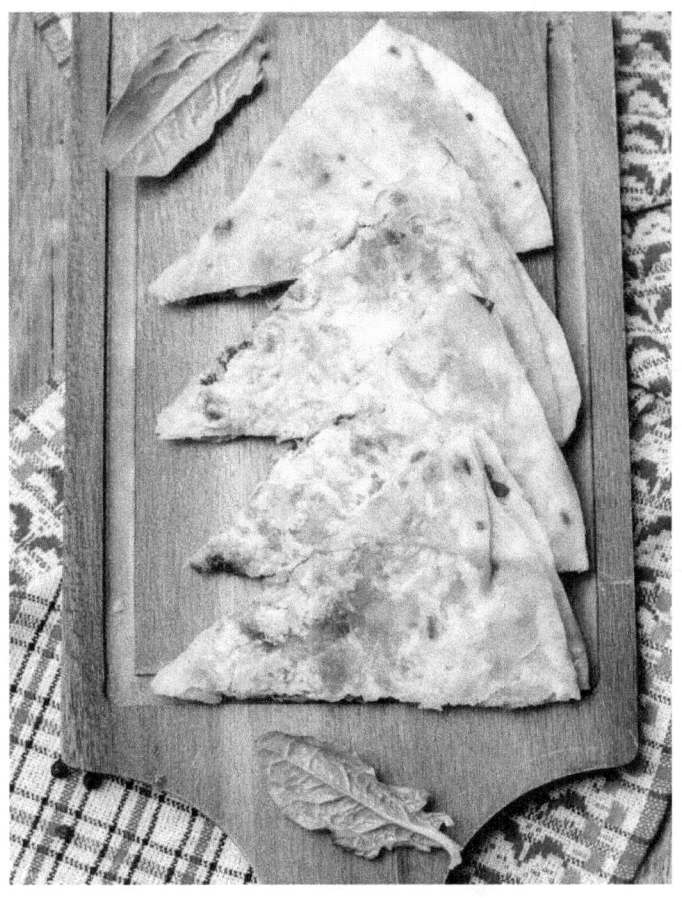

Preparation Time: 10minutes

Cooking Time: 20minutes

Serving: 4

Ingredients:

Tortillas

- 3 tbsp flax seed powder + ½ cup water
- ½ cup dairy-free cashew cream
- 1 tbsp coconut flour
- 1½ tsp psyllium husk powder
- ½ tsp salt

Filling

- 5 oz. grated cheddar cheese
- 1 tbsp cashew butter, for frying
- 1 oz. leafy greens

Directions:

1. Preheat the oven to 400 °F.
2. In a bowl, mix the flax seed powder with water and allow sitting to thicken for 5 minutes.
3. After, whisk the cashew cream into the flax egg until the batter is smooth.
4. In another bowl, combine the psyllium husk powder, coconut flour, and salt. Add the flour mixture to the flax egg batter and fold in until fully incorporated. Allow sitting for a few minutes.

5. Then, line a baking sheet with parchment paper and pour in the mixture. Spread into the baking sheet using a spatula and bake in the oven's upper rack for 5 to 7 minutes or until brown around the edges. Keep a watchful eye on the tortillas to prevent burning.
6. Remove when ready and slice into 8 pieces. Set aside.
7. For the filling, spoon a little cashew butter into a skillet and place a tortilla in the pan. Sprinkle with some cheddar cheese, leafy greens, and cover with another tortilla.
8. Brown each side of the quesadilla for 1 minute or until the cheese melts. Transfer to a plate.
9. Repeat assembling the quesadillas using the remaining cashew butter.
10. Serve immediately with avocado salad.

Nutrition:

Calories:224, Total Fat:20.4g, Saturated Fat:12.2g, Total Carbs: 1g, Dietary Fiber:0g, Sugar:1g, Protein:9g, Sodium:556mg

Grapes and Tomato Salad

Preparation time: 10 minutes

Cooking time: 0 minutes

Servings: 4

Ingredients:

- 1 pound cherry tomatoes, halved
- 2 cups green grapes, halved
- 2 tablespoons olive oil
- 4 spring onions, chopped
- 1 teaspoon cumin, ground
- 1 teaspoon rosemary, dried
- 1 tablespoon balsamic vinegar
- 1 tablespoon chives, chopped

Directions:

1. In a bowl, combine the grapes with the tomatoes and the other ingredients, toss and serve as a side salad.

Nutrition:

calories 140, fat 4, fiber 6, carbs 3.4, protein 4

Spinach Mix

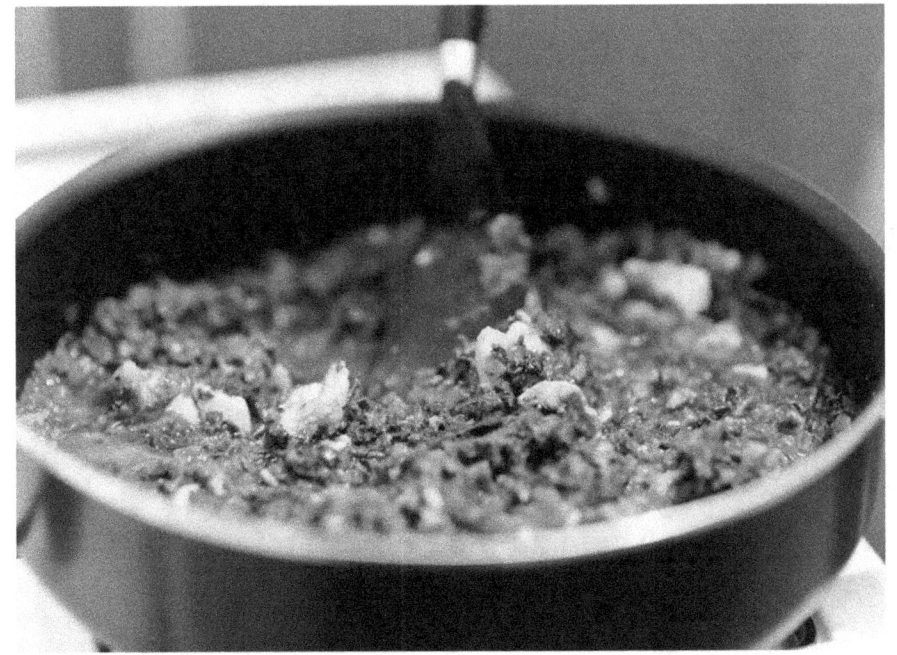

Preparation time: 10 minutes

Cooking time: 12 minutes

Servings: 4

Ingredients:

- 1 pound baby spinach
- 1 yellow onion, chopped
- 1 tablespoon lemon juice

- 1 tablespoon olive oil
- 2 garlic cloves, minced
- A pinch of cayenne pepper
- ¼ teaspoon smoked paprika
- A pinch of salt and black pepper

Directions:

1. Heat up a pan with the oil over medium-high heat, add the onion and the garlic and sauté for 2 minutes.
2. Add the spinach and the other ingredients, toss, cook over medium heat for 10 minutes, divide between plates and serve as a side dish.

Nutrition:

calories 71, fat 4, fiber 3.2, carbs 7.4, protein 3.7

Balsamic Brussels Sprouts

Preparation time: 10 minutes

Cooking time: 20 minutes

Servings: 4

Ingredients:

- 2 pounds Brussels sprouts, trimmed and halved
- 1 tablespoon avocado oil
- 2 tablespoons balsamic vinegar
- 3 garlic cloves, minced
- 1 tablespoon cilantro, chopped
- A pinch of salt and black pepper

Directions:

1. Heat up a pan with the oil over medium-high heat, add the garlic and sauté for 2 minutes.
2. Add the sprouts and the other ingredients, toss, cook over medium heat for 18 minutes more, divide between plates and serve.

Nutrition:

calories 108, fat 1.2, fiber 8.7, carbs 21.7, protein 7.9

Chili Asparagus

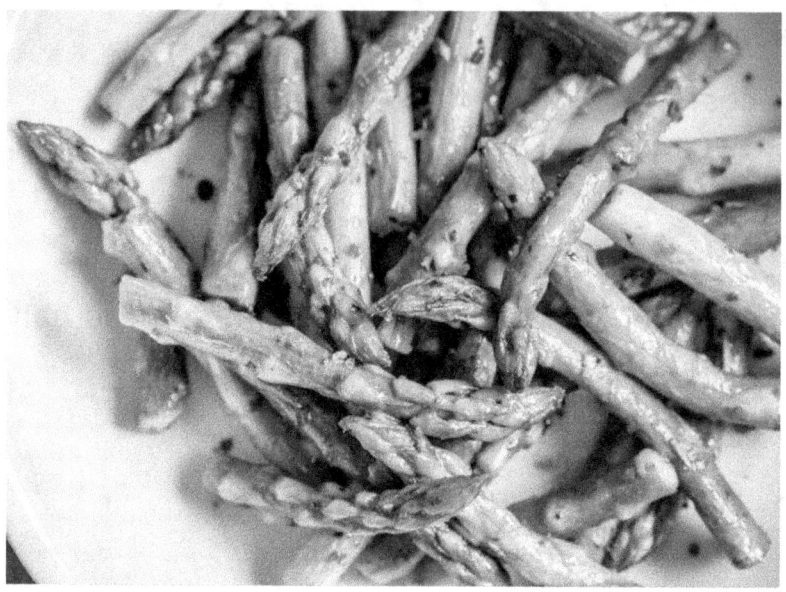

Preparation time: 10 minutes

Cooking time: 15 minutes

Servings: 4

Ingredients:

- 1 bunch asparagus, trimmed and halved
- 1 yellow onion, chopped
- 2 tablespoons olive oil
- 2 garlic cloves, minced

- 1 teaspoon chili powder
- ¼ cup cilantro, chopped

Directions:

1. Heat up a pan with the oil over medium-high heat, add the onion and the garlic and sauté for 5 minutes.
2. Add the asparagus and the other ingredients, toss, cook for 10 minutes, divide between plates and serve.

Nutrition:

calories 80, fat 7.2, fiber 1.4, carbs 4.4, protein 1

Sweet Potato Mash

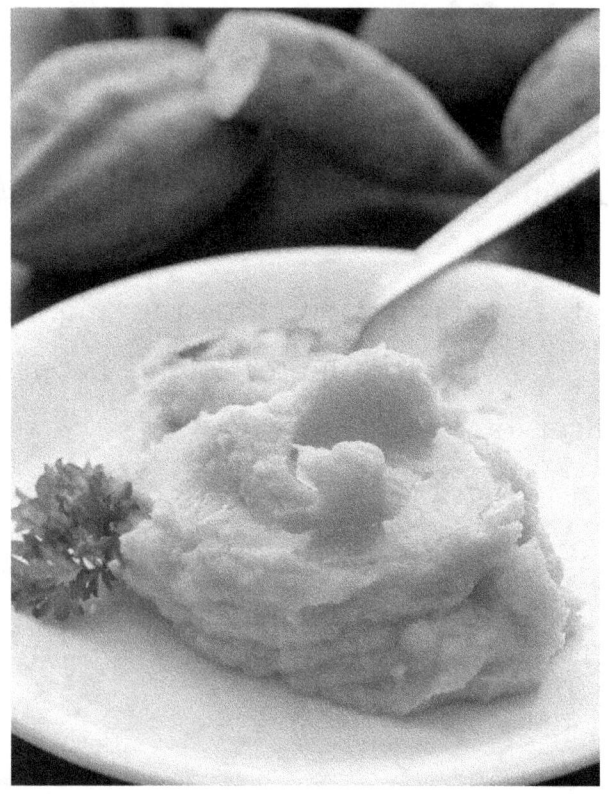

Preparation time: 10 minutes

Cooking time: 25 minutes

Servings: 4

Ingredients:

- 1 pound sweet potatoes, peeled and cubed
- 1 cup veggie stock
- 1 cup coconut cream
- 2 teaspoons olive oil
- A pinch of salt and black pepper
- ½ teaspoon turmeric powder
- 1 tablespoon chives, chopped

Directions:

1. In a pot, combine the stock with the sweet potatoes and the other ingredients except the cream, the oil and the chives, stir, bring to a simmer and cook over medium heat for 25 minutes.
2. Add the rest of the ingredients, mash the mix well, stir it, divide between plates and serve.

Nutrition:

calories 200, fat 4, fiber 4, carbs 7, protein 10

Simple Potatoes Side Dish

Preparation time: 10 minutes

Cooking time: 3 hours

Servings: 12

Ingredients:

- 2 tablespoons olive oil
- 3 pounds new potatoes, halved
- 7 garlic cloves, minced
- 1 tablespoon rosemary, chopped
- A pinch of salt and black pepper

Directions:

1. In your slow cooker, mix oil with potatoes, garlic, rosemary, salt and pepper, toss, cover and cook on High for 3 hours.
2. Divide between plates and serve as a side dish.
3. Enjoy!

Nutrition:

calories 102, fat 2, fiber 2, carbs 18, protein 2

Special Potatoes Mix

Preparation time: 10 minutes

Cooking time: 7 hours

Servings: 10

Ingredients:

- 2 green apples, cored and cut into wedges
- 3 pounds sweet potatoes, peeled and cut into medium wedges
- ½ cup dried cherries
- 1 cup coconut cream
- 1 cup apple butter
- 1 and ½ teaspoon pumpkin pie spice

Directions:

1. In your slow cooker, mix sweet potatoes with green apples, cream, cherries, apple butter and spice, toss, cover and cook on Low for 7 hours.
2. Toss, divide between plates and serve as a side dish.
3. Enjoy!

Nutrition:

calories 351, fat 8, fiber 5, carbs 48, protein 2

Cumin Cauliflower Rice and Broccoli

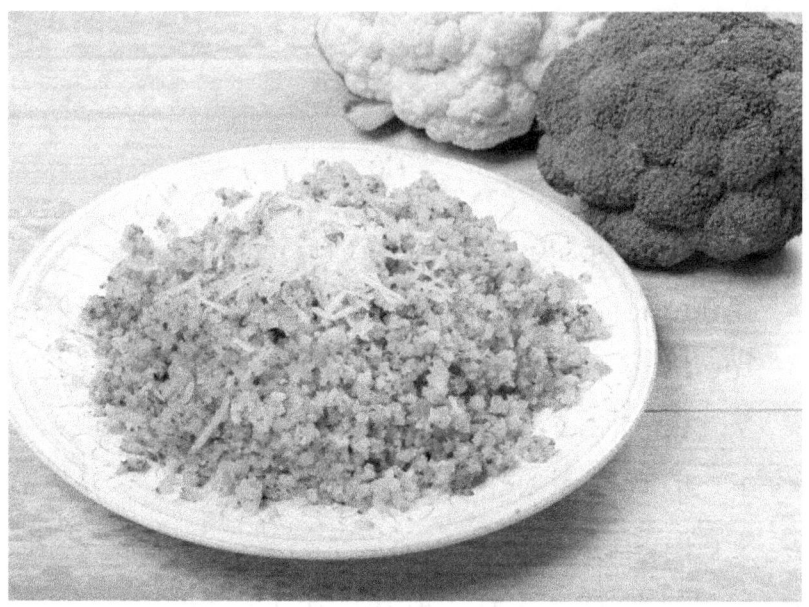

Preparation time: 10 minutes

Cooking time: 25 minutes

Servings: 4

Ingredients:

- 2 cups cauliflower rice
- 1 cup broccoli florets
- 2 tablespoons olive oil
- 4 scallions, chopped
- 1 teaspoon sweet paprika

- 1 teaspoon chili powder
- 1 cup vegetable stock
- 1 teaspoon red pepper flakes
- A pinch of salt and black pepper
- ¼ teaspoon cumin, ground

Directions:

1. Heat up a pan with the oil over medium heat, add the scallions, paprika and chili powder and sauté for 5 minutes.
2. Add the cauliflower rice and the other ingredients, toss, bring to a simmer, cook over medium heat for 20 minutes, divide between plates and serve.

Nutrition:

calories 81, fat 7.9, fiber 1.5, carbs 4.1, protein 1.1

Radish and Broccoli

Preparation time: 10 minutes

Cooking time: 30 minutes

Servings: 4

Ingredients:

- 2 tablespoons olive oil
- 1 pound broccoli florets
- 4 scallions, chopped
- ½ pound radishes, halved
- 4 garlic cloves, minced
- 2 teaspoons cumin, ground
- 2 tablespoons tomato passata
- ½ cup veggie stock
- A pinch of salt and black pepper

Directions:

1. Heat up a pan with the oil over medium heat, add the scallions and sauté for 5 minutes.
2. Add the broccoli, radishes and the other ingredients, toss, cook over medium heat for 25 minutes more, divide between plates and serve.

Nutrition:

calories 261, fat 5, fiber 4, carbs 9, protein 12

Mashed Broccoli

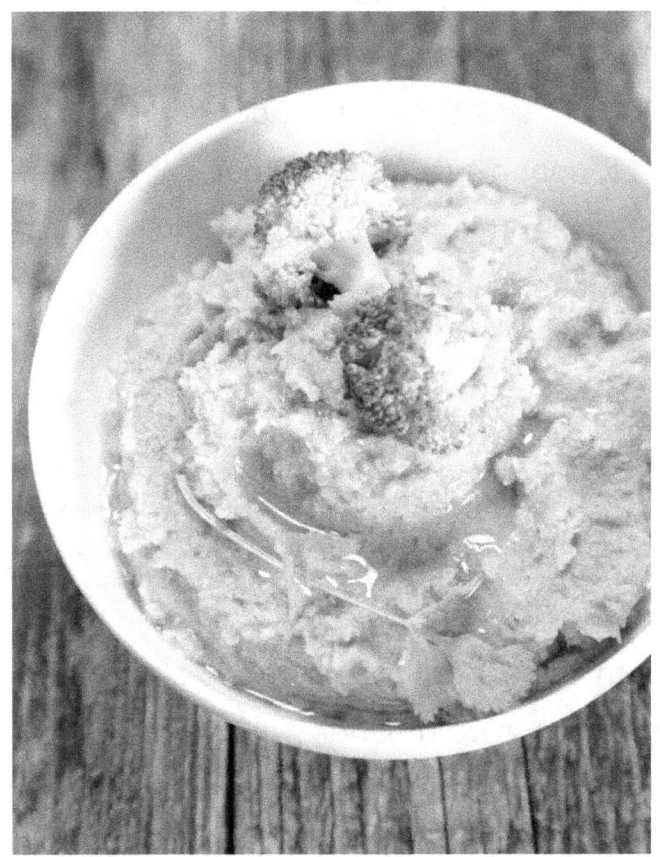

Preparation time: 10 minutes

Cooking time: 25 minutes

Servings: 4

Ingredients:

- 1 and ½ cups water
- 1 pound broccoli florets
- 2 teaspoons olive oil
- A pinch of salt and black pepper
- ½ teaspoon turmeric powder
- ½ teaspoon cumin, ground
- 1 tablespoon chives, chopped

Directions:

1. Put the water in a pot, add the broccoli, salt and pepper, bring to a boil and cook over medium heat for 25 minutes.
2. Drain the broccoli, transfer to a bowl, and mash using a potato masher.
3. Add the rest of the ingredients, mash everything again, stir as well, divide between plates and serve as a side dish.

Nutrition:

calories 200, fat 4, fiber 4, carbs 7, protein 10

Roasted Cauliflower Tacos

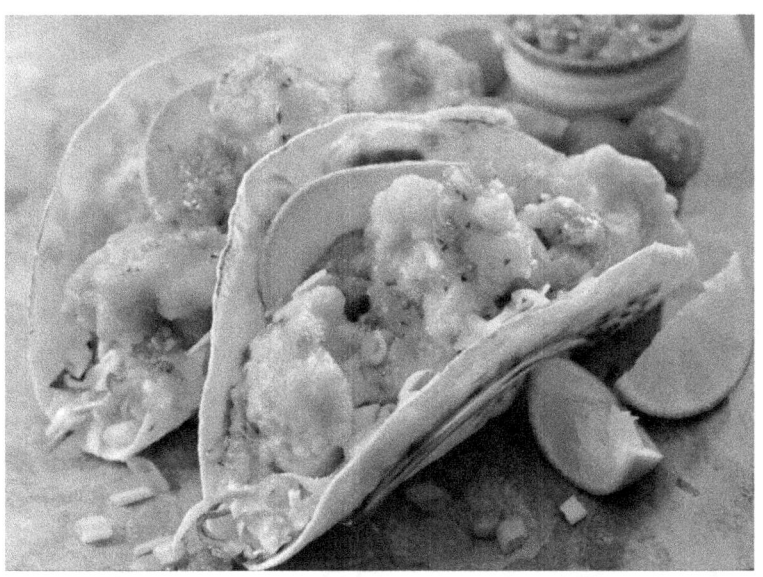

Preparation time: 10 minutes

cooking time: 30 minutes

Servings: 8 TACOS

Ingredients

For the roasted cauliflower

- 1 head cauliflower, cut into bite-size pieces
- 1 tablespoon olive oil (optional
- 2 tablespoons whole-wheat flour

- 2 tablespoons nutritional yeast
- 1 to 2 teaspoons smoked paprika
- ½ to 1 teaspoon chili powder
- Pinch sea salt

For the tacos

- 2 cups shredded lettuce
- 2 cups cherry tomatoes, quartered
- 2 carrots, scrubbed or peeled, and grated
- ½ cup Fresh Mango Salsa
- ½ cup Guacamole
- 8 small whole-grain or corn tortillas
- 1 lime, cut into 8 wedges

Directions

To Make The Roasted Cauliflower

1. Preheat the oven to 350 °F. Lightly grease a large rectangular baking sheet with olive oil, or line it with parchment paper. In a large bowl, toss the cauliflower pieces with oil (if using), or just rinse them so they're wet. The idea is to get the seasonings to stick. In a smaller bowl, mix together the flour, nutritional yeast, paprika, chili powder, and salt.

2. Add the seasonings to the cauliflower, and mix it around with your hands to thoroughly coat. Spread the cauliflower on the baking sheet, and roast for 20 to 30 minutes, or until softened.

To Make The Tacos.

3. Prep the veggies, salsa, and guacamole while the cauliflower is roasting. Once the cauliflower is cooked, heat the tortillas for just a few minutes in the oven or in a small skillet. Set everything out on the table, and assemble your tacos as you go. Give a squeeze of fresh lime just before eating.

Nutrition (1 taco):

Calories: 198; Total fat: 6g; Carbs: 32g; Fiber: 6g; Protein: 7g

Creamy Mint-Lime Spaghetti Squash

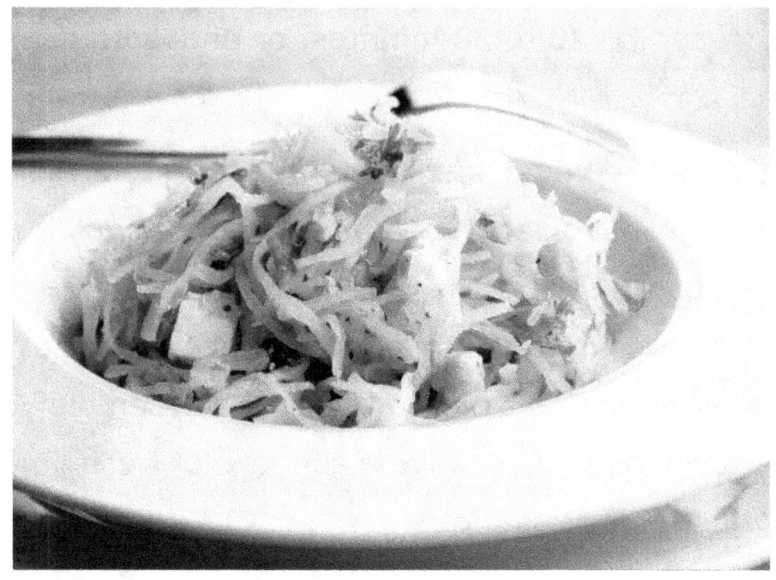

Preparation time: 10 minutes

cooking time: 30 minutes

servings: 3

Ingredients

For the dressing

- 3 tablespoons tahini
- Zest and juice of 1 small lime

- 2 tablespoons fresh mint, minced
- 1 small garlic clove, pressed
- 1 tablespoon nutritional yeast
- Pinch sea salt

For the spaghetti squash

- 1 spaghetti squash
- Pinch sea salt
- 1 cup cherry tomatoes, chopped
- 1 cup chopped bell pepper, any color
- Freshly ground black pepper

Directions

To Make The Dressing

1. Make the dressing by whisking together the tahini and lime juice until thick, stirring in water if you need it, until smooth, then add the rest of the ingredients. Or you can purée all the ingredients in a blender.

To Make The Spaghetti Squash.

2. Put a large pot of water on high and bring to a boil. Cut the squash in half and scoop out the seeds. Put the squash halves in the pot with the salt, and boil for about 30 minutes. Carefully

remove the squash from the pot and let it cool until you can safely handle it. Set half the squash aside for another meal. Scoop out the squash from the skin, which stays hard like a shell, and break the strands apart. The flesh absorbs water while boiling, so set the "noodles" in a strainer for 10 minutes, tossing occasionally to drain. Transfer the cooked spaghetti squash to a large bowl and toss with the mint-lime dressing. Then top with the cherry tomatoes and bell pepper. Add an extra sprinkle of nutritional yeast and black pepper, if you wish.

Nutrition:

Calories: 199; Total fat: 10g; Carbs: 27g; Fiber: 5g; Protein: 7g

Marsala Carrots

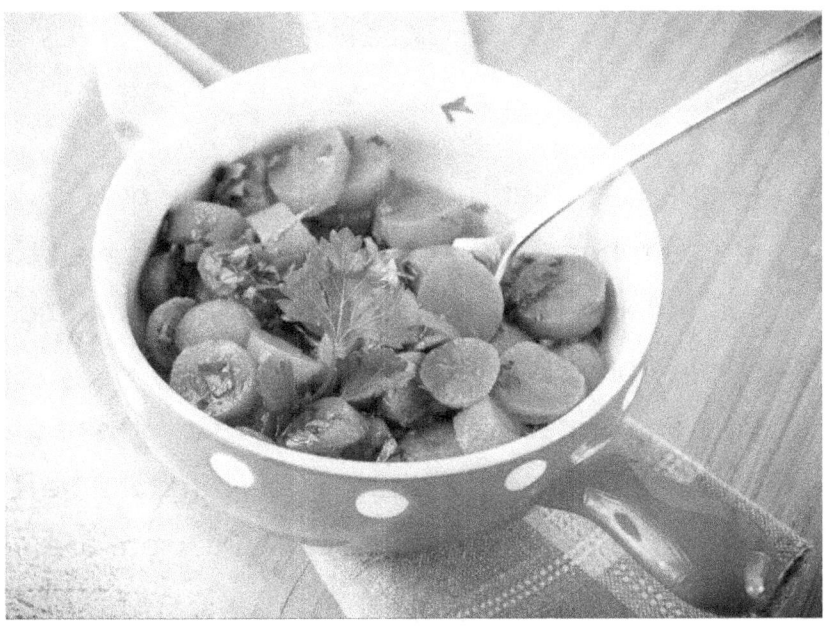

Preparation time: 5 minutes

cooking time: 20 minutes

servings: 4

Ingredients

- 2 tablespoons vegan margarine
- 1 pound carrots, cut diagonally into 1/4-inch slices
- Salt and freshly ground black pepper

- 1/2 cup Marsala
- 1/4 cup water
- 1/4 cup chopped fresh parsley, for garnish

Directions

1. In a large skillet, melt the margarine over medium heat. Add the carrots and toss well to coat evenly with the margarine. Cover and cook, stirring occasionally, for 5 minutes.
2. Season with salt and pepper to taste, tossing to coat. Add the Marsala and water. Reduce heat to low, cover, and simmer until the carrots are tender, about 15 minutes.
3. Uncover and cook over medium-high heat until the liquid is reduced into a syrupy sauce, stirring to prevent burning.
4. Transfer to a serving bowl and sprinkle with parsley. Serve immediately.

Garlic And Herb Zoodles

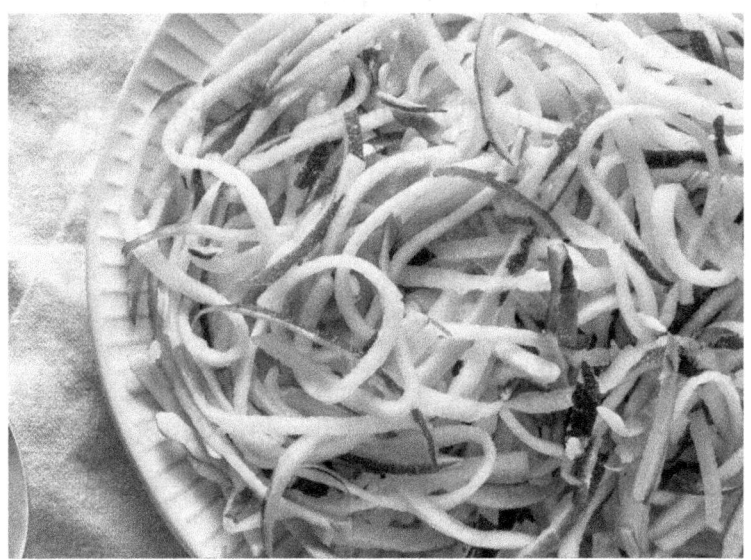

Preparation time: 10 minutes

cooking time: 2 minutes

servings: 4

Ingredients

- 1 teaspoon extra-virgin olive oil or 2 tablespoons vegetable broth
- 1 teaspoon minced garlic (about 1 clove
- 4 medium zucchini, spiralized

- ½ teaspoon dried oregano
- ½ teaspoon dried basil
- ¼ to ½ teaspoon red pepper flakes, to taste
- ¼ teaspoon salt (optional
- ¼ teaspoon freshly ground black pepper

Directions

1. In a large skillet over medium-high heat, heat the olive oil.
2. Add the garlic, zucchini, basil, oregano, red pepper flakes, salt (if using), and black pepper. Sauté for 1 to 2 minutes, until barely tender. Divide the zoodles evenly among 4 storage containers. Let cool before sealing the lids.

Nutrition:

Calories: 44; Fat: 2g; Protein: 3g; Carbohydrates: 7g; Fiber: 2g; Sugar: 3g; Sodium: 20mg

Artichokes and Mushroom Mix

Preparation time: 30 minutes

Cooking time: 30 minutes

Servings: 4

Ingredients:

- 16 mushrooms, sliced
- 1/3 cup tamari sauce
- 4 tablespoons balsamic vinegar
- 1/3 cup olive oil
- 4 garlic cloves, minced
- 1 tablespoon lemon juice
- 1 teaspoon oregano, dried
- 1 teaspoon rosemary, dried
- ½ tablespoon thyme, dried
- Black pepper to taste
- 1 sweet onion, chopped
- A pinch of sea salt
- 1 jar artichoke hearts
- 4 cups spinach
- 1 tablespoon coconut oil

- 1 teaspoon garlic powder
- 1 teaspoon garlic, minced
- 1 cauliflower head, florets separated
- ½ cup veggie stock
- A pinch of nutmeg, ground

Directions:

1. In a bowl, mix vinegar with tamari sauce, lemon juice, 4 garlic cloves, olive oil, oregano, rosemary, thyme, a pinch of salt, black pepper and mushrooms, toss to coat well and leave aside for 30 minutes.
2. Transfer these to a lined baking sheet and bake them in the oven at 350 degrees F for 30 minutes.
3. In a food processor, mix cauliflower with a pinch of sea salt and black pepper and pulse until you obtain rice.
4. Heat a pan to medium-high heat, add cauliflower rice, toast for 2 minutes, add nutmeg, garlic powder, black pepper and stock, stir and cook until stock evaporated.

5. Heat a pan with the coconut oil over medium heat, add onion, artichokes, 1 teaspoon garlic and spinach, stir and cook for a few minutes.
6. Divide cauliflower rice on plates, top with artichokes and mushrooms and serve.

Nutritional value/serving:

calories 354, fat 29,9, fiber 4,3, carbs 16,5, protein 6,6

Orange Juice Smoothie

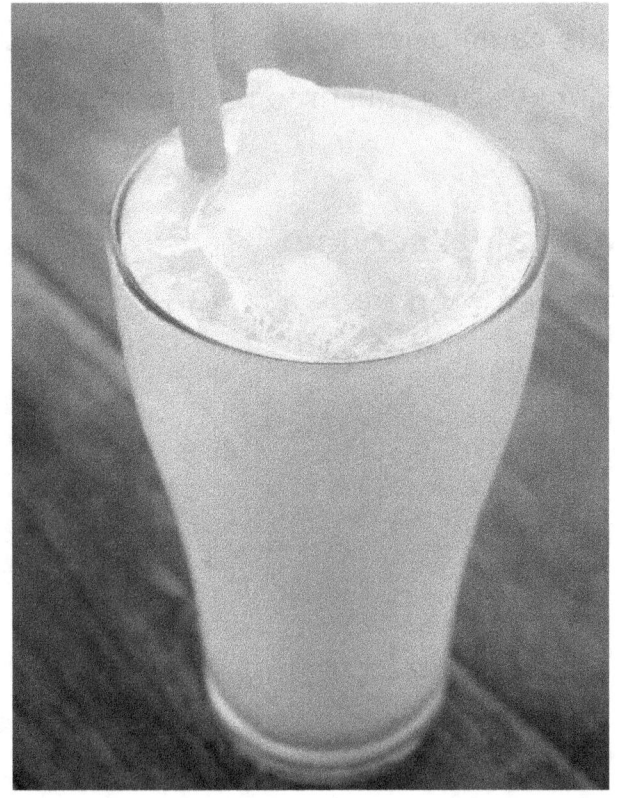

Preparation Time: 5 mins

Servings: 2

Ingredients:

- ¼ c. frozen orange juice concentrate

- 1 c. fat-free vanilla frozen yogurt
- ¾ c. fat-free milk

Directions:

1. Add the ingredients to a blender and pulse until they are smooth.
2. Pour them into frosted glasses and serve.

Nutrition:

Calories: 180, Fat:0 g, Carbs:38 g, Protein:7 g, Sugars:20 g, Sodium:5 mg

Vegan Rice Pudding

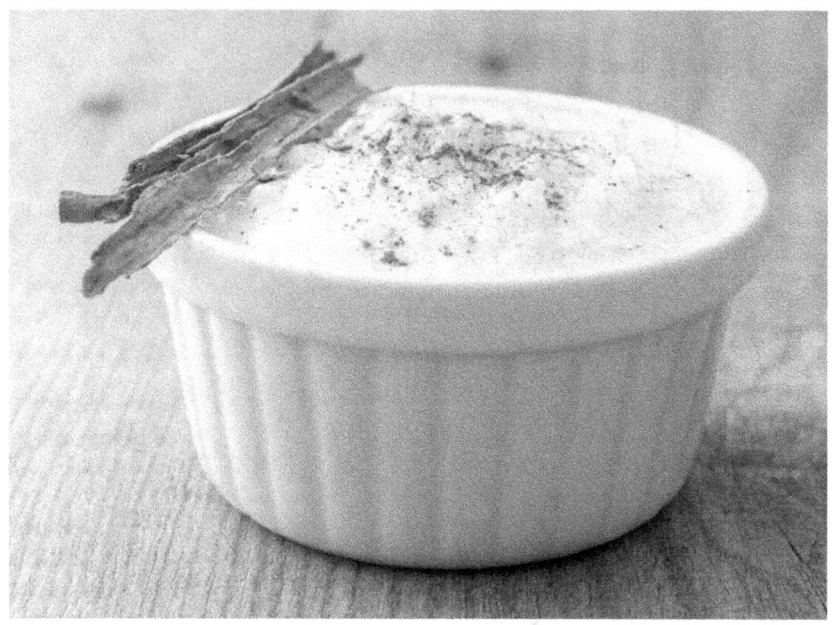

Preparation Time: 5 mins

Servings: 8

Ingredients:

- ½ tsp. ground cinnamon
- 1 c. rinsed basmati
- ¼ c. sugar
- 1/8 tsp. ground cardamom

- 1/8 tsp. pure almond extract
- 1 quart vanilla nondairy milk
- 1 tsp. pure vanilla extract

Directions:

1. Measure all of the ingredients into a saucepan and stir well to combine. Bring to a boil over medium-high heat.
2. Once boiling, reduce heat to low and simmer, stirring very frequently, about 15–20 minutes.
3. Remove from heat and cool. Serve sprinkled with additional ground cinnamon if desired.

Nutrition:

Calories: 148, Fat:2 g, Carbs:26 g, Protein:4 g, Sugars:35 g, Sodium:150 mg

Asparagus Frittata

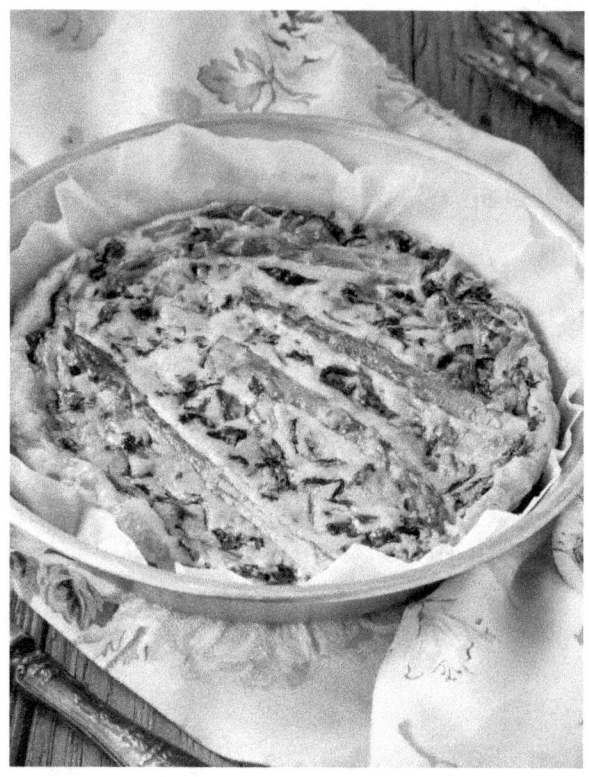

Preparation time: 10 minutes

Cooking time: 15 minutes

Servings: 4

Ingredients:

- 4 eggs, whisked
- ¼ cup onion, chopped
- A drizzle of olive oil
- 1 pound asparagus spears, cut into 1-inch pieces
- Salt and ground black pepper, to taste
- 1 cup cheddar cheese, grated

Directions:

1. Heat up a pan with the oil over medium-high heat, add the onions, stir, and cook for 3 minutes.
2. Add the asparagus, stir, and cook for 6 minutes.
3. Add the eggs, stir, and cook for 3 minutes.
4. Add the salt and pepper, sprinkle with the cheese, place in an oven, and broil for 3 minutes.
5. Divide the frittata on plates and serve.

Nutrition:

Calories - 200, Fat - 12, Fiber - 2, Carbs - 5, Protein - 14

Mushroom & Wild Rice Stew

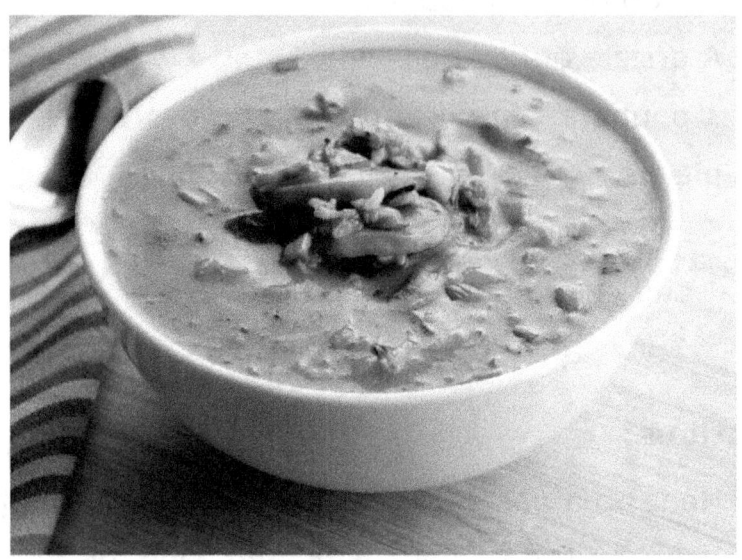

Preparation time: 10 minutes

cooking time: 50 minutes

servings: 6

Ingredients

- 1 to 2 teaspoons olive oil
- 2 cups chopped mushrooms
- ½ to 1 teaspoon salt
- 1 onion, chopped, or 1 teaspoon onion powder

- 3 or 4 garlic cloves, minced, or ½ teaspoon garlic powder
- 1 tablespoon dried herbs
- ¾ cup brown rice
- ¼ cup wild rice or additional brown rice
- 3 cups water
- 3 cups Economical Vegetable Broth or store-bought broth
- 2 to 4 tablespoons balsamic vinegar (optional
- Freshly ground black pepper
- 1 cup frozen peas, thawed
- 1 cup unsweetened nondairy milk (optional
- 1 to 2 cups chopped greens, such as spinach, kale, or chard

Directions

1. Heat the olive oil in a large soup pot over medium-high heat.
2. Add the mushrooms and a pinch of salt, and sauté for about 4 minutes, until the mushrooms are softened. Add the onion and garlic (if using fresh), and sauté for 1 to 2 minutes more. Stir in the dried herbs (plus the onion powder and/or garlic powder, if using), white or brown rice,

wild rice, water, vegetable broth, vinegar (if using), and salt and pepper to taste. Bring to a boil, turn the heat to low, and cover the pot. Simmer the soup for 15 minutes (for white rice) or 45 minutes (for brown rice). Turn off the heat and stir in the peas, milk (if using), and greens. Let the greens wilt before serving.
3. Leftovers will keep in an airtight container for up to 1 week in the refrigerator or up to 1 month in the freezer.

Nutrition (2 cups)

Calories: 201; Protein: 6g; Total fat: 3g; Saturated fat: 0g; Carbohydrates: 44g; Fiber: 4g

Tamarind Chickpea Stew

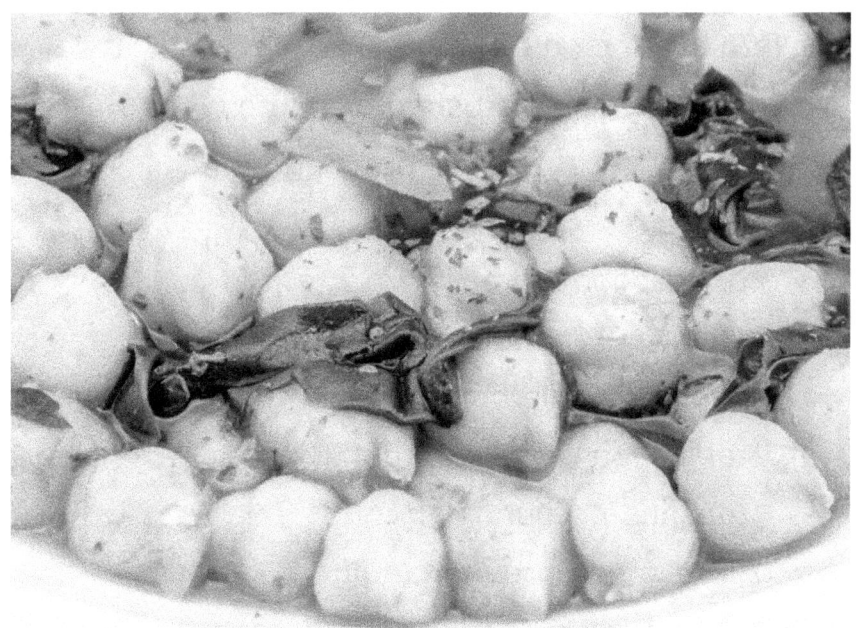

Preparation time: 5 minutes

cooking time: 60 minutes

servings: 4

Ingredients

- 1 tablespoon olive oil
- 1 large onion, chopped

- 3 cups cooked chickpeas or 2 (15.5-ouncecans chickpeas, drained and rinsed
- 2 medium Yukon Gold potatoes, peeled and cut into 1/4-inch dice
- 1 (28-ouncecan crushed tomatoes
- 1 (4-ouncecan mild chopped green chiles, drained
- 2 tablespoons tamarind paste
- 1/4 cup pure maple syrup
- 1 cup vegetable broth, homemade or water
- 2 tablespoons chili powder
- 1 teaspoon ground coriander
- 1/2 teaspoon ground cumin
- Salt and freshly ground black pepper
- 1 cup frozen baby peas, thawed

Directions

1. In a large saucepan, heat the oil over medium heat. Add the onion, cover, and cook until softened, about 5 minutes. Add the potatoes, chickpeas, tomatoes, and chiles and simmer, uncovered, for 5 minutes.

2. In a small bowl, combine the tamarind paste, maple syrup, and broth and blend until smooth. Stir the tamarind mixture into the vegetables, along with the chili powder, coriander, cumin, and salt and pepper to taste. Bring to a boil, then reduce the heat to medium and simmer, covered, until the potatoes are tender, about 40 minutes.
3. Taste, adjusting seasonings if necessary, and stir in the peas. Simmer, uncovered, about 10 minutes longer. Serve immediately.

Pesto Parmesan Tempeh with Green Pasta

Preparation Time: 1 hour 27 minutes

Serving: 4

Ingredients:

- 4 tempeh
- 1 tbsp butter
- 4 large turnips, Blade C, noodle trimmed
- ½ cup basil pesto, olive oil-based
- 1 cup grated parmesan cheese
- Salt and black pepper to taste

Directions:

1. Preheat the oven to 350 °F.
2. Season the tempeh with salt, black pepper and place on a baking sheet. Divide the pesto on top and spread well on the tempeh.
3. Place the sheet in the oven and bake for 45 minutes to 1 hour or until cooked through.

4. When ready, pull out the baking sheet and divide half of the parmesan cheese on top of the tempeh. Cook further for 10 minutes or until the cheese melts. Remove the tempeh and set aside for serving.
5. Melt the butter in a medium skillet and sauté the turnips until tender, 5 to 7 minutes. Stir in the remaining parmesan cheese and divide between serving plates.
6. Top with the tempeh and serve warm.

Nutrition:

Calories:442, Total Fat:29.4g, Saturated Fat:11.3g, Total Carbs:8g, Dietary Fiber:1g, Sugar:1g, Protein:39g, Sodium:814mg

Creamy Tofu with Green Beans and Keto Fettuccine

Preparation Time: 40 minutes + overtime chilling time

Serving size: 4

Ingredients:

For the keto fettuccine:

- 1 egg yolk
- 1 cup shredded mozzarella cheese

For the creamy tofu and green beans:

- 1 tbsp olive oil
- ½ cup green beans, chopped
- 4 tofu, cut into thin strips
- Salt and black pepper to taste
- 1 lemon, zested and juiced
- ¼ cup vegetable broth
- 1 cup plain yogurt
- 6 basil leaves, chopped
- 1 cup shaved parmesan cheese for topping

Directions:

For the keto fettucine:

1. Pour the cheese into a medium safe-microwave bowl and melt in the microwave for 35 minutes or until melted.
2. Take out the bowl and allow cooling for 1 minute only to warm the cheese but not cool completely. Mix in the egg yolk until well-combined.
3. Lay a parchment paper on a flat surface, pour the cheese mixture on top and cover with another parchment paper. Using a rolling pin, flatten the dough into 1/8-inch thickness.
4. Take off the parchment paper and cut the dough into thick fettuccine strands. Place in a bowl and refrigerate overnight.
5. When ready to cook, bring 2 cups of water to a boil in medium saucepan and add the keto fettuccine. Cook for 40 seconds to 1 minute and then drain through a colander. Run cold water over the pasta and set aside to cool.

For the creamy tofu and green beans:

6. Heat the olive oil in a large skillet, season the tofu with salt, black pepper, and cook in the oil

until brown on the outside and slightly cooked through, 10 minutes.
7. Mix in the green beans and cook until softened, 5 minutes.
8. Stir in the lemon zest, lemon juice, and vegetable broth. Cook for 5 more minutes or until the liquid reduces by a quarter.
9. Add the plain yogurt and mix well. Pour in the keto fettuccine and basil, fold in well and cook for 1 minute. Adjust the taste with salt and black pepper as desired.
10. Dish the food onto serving plates, top with the parmesan cheese and serve warm.

Nutrition:

Calories:721, Total Fat:76.8g, Saturated Fat:21.2g, Total Carbs:2g, Dietary Fiber:0g, Sugar:0g, Protein:9g, Sodium:309mg

Rice Salad With Cashews And Dried Papaya

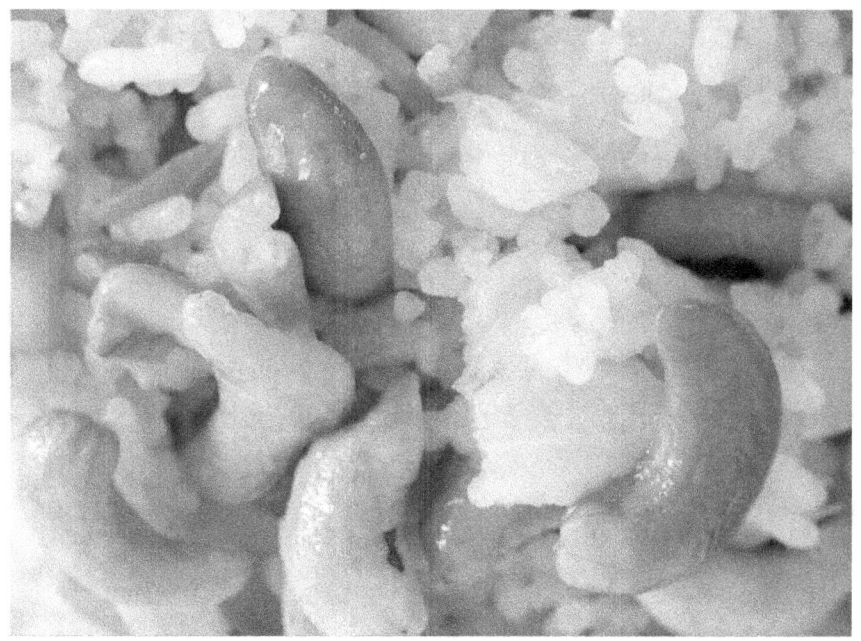

Preparation time: 15 minutes

cooking time: 0 minutes

servings: 4

Ingredients

- 31/2 cups cooked brown rice
- 1/2 cup chopped roasted cashews

- 1/2 cup thinly sliced dried papaya
- 2 teaspoons agave nectar
- 4 green onions, chopped
- 3 tablespoons fresh lime juice
- 1 teaspoon grated fresh ginger
- 1/3 cup grapeseed oil
- Salt and freshly ground black pepper

Directions

1. In a large bowl, combine the rice, cashews, papaya, and green onions. Set aside.
2. In a small bowl, combine the lime juice, agave nectar, and ginger. Whisk in the oil and season with the salt and pepper to taste. Pour the dressing over the rice mixture, mix well, and serve.

Easy Avocado and Cremini Mushroom Melts

Preparation Time: 15 minutes

Cooking Time: 25 minutes

Servings: 4

Ingredients:

- 8 sliced Cremini mushrooms
- 1 tbsp. olive oil
- 3 slices Keto bread
- 1 c. guacamole
- 1 tbsp. balsamic vinegar
- 12 slices cheddar cheese
- Salt
- Pepper

Directions:

1. Preheat oven to 350 °F.
2. Using a skillet, Sauté balsamic vinegar, mushrooms, and olive oil medium-high heat for 15 minutes, as you stir often, until mushrooms are fragrant and golden brown.

3. Spread guacamole on bread and top with sautéed cheese and mushrooms.
4. Bake for approximately 10 minutes and ensure all the cheese melts out.
5. Serve and enjoy!

Nutrition:

Calories: 77, Fat: 16.25g, Carbs: 11.35g, Protein: 9.32g

Potato Chips

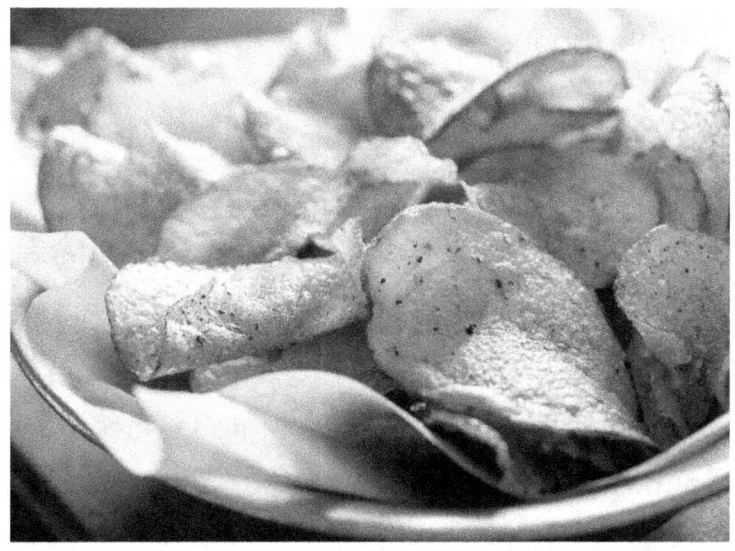

Preparation Time: 10 minutes

Cooking Time: 20 minutes

Servings: 2

Ingredients:

- 3 medium potatoes, scrubbed, thinly sliced, soaked in warm water for 10 min
- ½ teaspoon onion powder
- ½ teaspoon red chili powder
- ½ teaspoon garlic powder

- ½ teaspoon curry powder
- 1 teaspoon of sea salt
- 1 tablespoon apple cider vinegar
- 2 tablespoons olive oil

Direction:

1. Drain the potato slices, pat dry, then place them in a large bowl, add remaining ingredients and toss until well coated.
2. Spread the potatoes in a single layer on a baking sheet and bake for 20 minutes until crispy, turning halfway.
3. Serve straight away.

Nutrition:

Calories: 600 Cal, Fat: 30 g, Carbs: 78 g, Protein: 9 g, Fiber: 23 g

Loaded Baked Potatoes

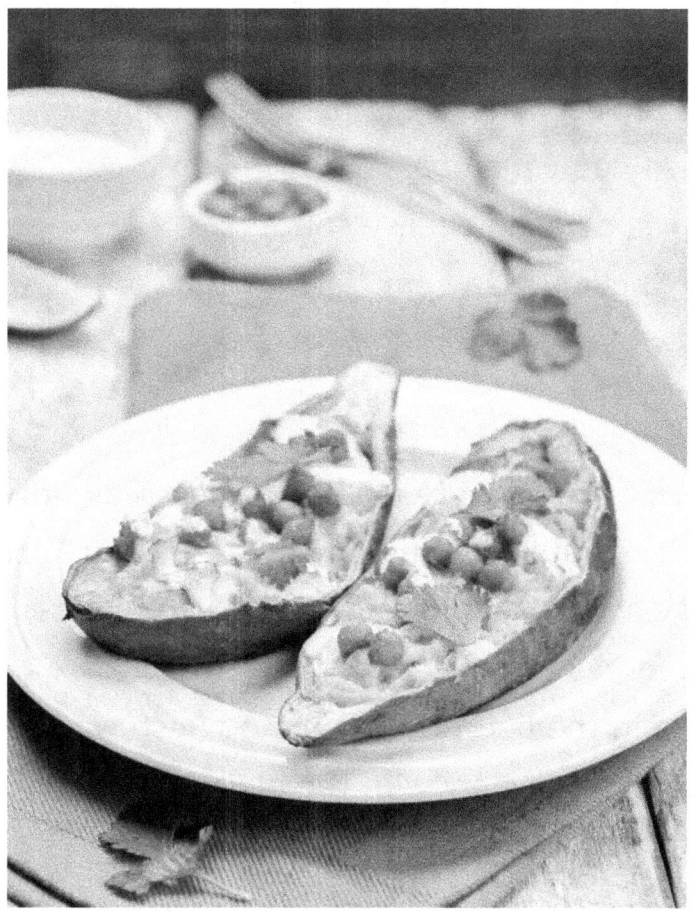

Preparation Time: 10 minutes

Cooking Time: 32 minutes

Servings: 2

Ingredients:

- 1/2 cup cooked chickpeas
- 2 medium potatoes, scrubbed
- 1 cup broccoli florets, steamed
- 2 tablespoons all-purpose seasoning
- 1/4 cup vegan bacon bits
- ¼ cup vegan cheese sauce
- 1/2 cup vegan sour cream

Directions:

1. Pierce hole in the potatoes, microwave them for 12 minutes over high heat setting until soft to touch and then bake them for 20 minutes at 450 degrees f until very tender.
2. Open the potatoes, mash the flesh with a fork, then top evenly with remaining ingredients and serve.

Nutrition:

Calories: 422 Cal, Fat: 16 g, Carbs: 59 g, Protein: 9 g, Fiber: 6 g

Almond Green Beans

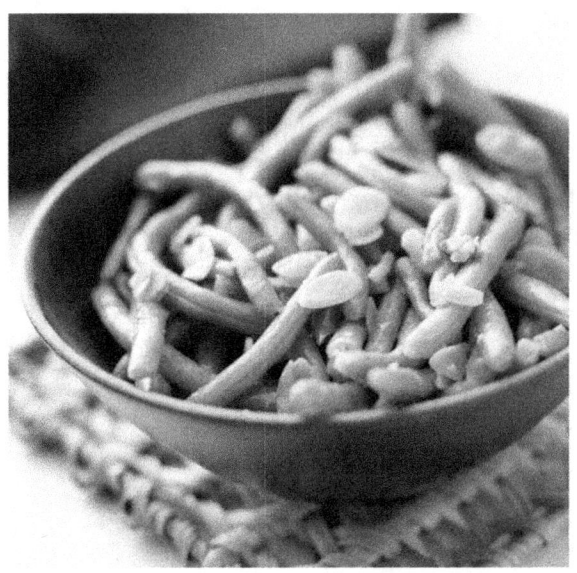

Preparation Time: 10 minutes

Cooking Time: 10 minutes

Servings: 4

Ingredients:

- 1 lb fresh green beans, trimmed
- 1/3 cup almonds, sliced
- 2 tbsp olive oil
- 1 tbsp lemon juice
- 4 garlic cloves, sliced

- ½ tsp sea salt

Directions:

1. Add green beans, salt, and lemon juice in a mixing bowl. Toss well and set aside.
2. Heat oil in a pan over medium heat.
3. Add sliced almonds and sauté until lightly browned.
4. Add garlic and sauté for 30 seconds.
5. Pour almond mixture over green beans and toss well.
6. Stir well and serve immediately.

Nutritions:

Calories 146 Fat 11.2 g Carbohydrates 10.9 g Sugar 2 g Protein 4 g Cholesterol 0 mg

Tomato Asparagus Salad

Preparation Time: 5 minutes

Cooking Time: 2 minutes

Servings: 4

Ingredients:

- 1/2 lb asparagus, trimmed and cut into pieces
- 8 oz cherry tomatoes, halved
- For Dressings:
- 1/4 tsp garlic and herb seasoning blend
- 1 tbsp vinegar
- 1 tbsp shallot, minced
- 1 garlic clove, minced
- 1 tbsp water
- 2 tbsp olive oil

Directions:

1. Add 1 tablespoon of water and asparagus in a heatproof bowl and cover with cling film and microwave for 2 minutes.
2. Remove asparagus from bowl and place into ice water until cool.

3. Add asparagus and tomatoes into a medium bowl.
4. In a small bowl, mix together all remaining ingredients and pour over vegetables.
5. Toss vegetables well and serve.

Nutritions:

Calories 85Fat 7.2 g Carbohydrates 5.1 g Sugar 2.6 g Protein 1.9 g Cholesterol 0 mg

Spinach Tomato Stir Fry

Preparation Time: 10 minutes

Cooking Time: 15 minutes

Servings: 2

Ingredients:

- 1/2 cup cherry tomatoes, cut in half
- 4 cups spinach
- 1/2 onion, sliced
- 1 garlic clove, diced
- 1/2 tsp lemon zest
- 2 tsp olive oil
- 6 button mushrooms, sliced
- Pepper
- Salt

Directions:

1. Heat olive oil in a pan over medium heat.
2. Add mushrooms and sauté for 3-4 minutes or until lightly browned.
3. Remove mushrooms to a plate and set aside.

4. Add onion and sauté for 2-3 minutes or until softened.
5. Add tomatoes, garlic and lemon zest, and season with pepper and salt. Cook for 2-3 minutes and lightly smashed tomatoes with a spatula.
6. Now add mushrooms and spinach and stir well and cook until spinach is wilted.
7. Season with salt and drizzle with lemon juice.
8. Serve and enjoy.

Nutritions:

Calories 104 Fat 7.1 g Carbohydrates 8.9 g Sugar 3.6 g Protein 4.3 g Cholesterol 5 mg

Jalapeno and Cilantro Hummus

Preparation Time: 5 minutes

Cooking Time: 0 minute

Servings: 4

Ingredients:

- ½ cup cilantro
- 1 1/2 cups chickpeas, cooked
- 1/2 of jalapeno pepper, sliced
- ½ teaspoon minced garlic
- 1 tablespoon lime juice
- 1/4 cup tahini
- ½ teaspoon salt
- ¼ water

Directions:

1. Place all the ingredients in a bowl and pulse for 2 minutes until smooth.
2. Tip the hummus in a bowl, drizzle with oil sprinkle with cilantro, and then serve.

Nutrition:

Calories: 137 Cal, Fat: 2.3 g, Carbs: 23.3 g, Protein: 7.3 g, Fiber: 6.6 g

Chocolate Coconut Brownies

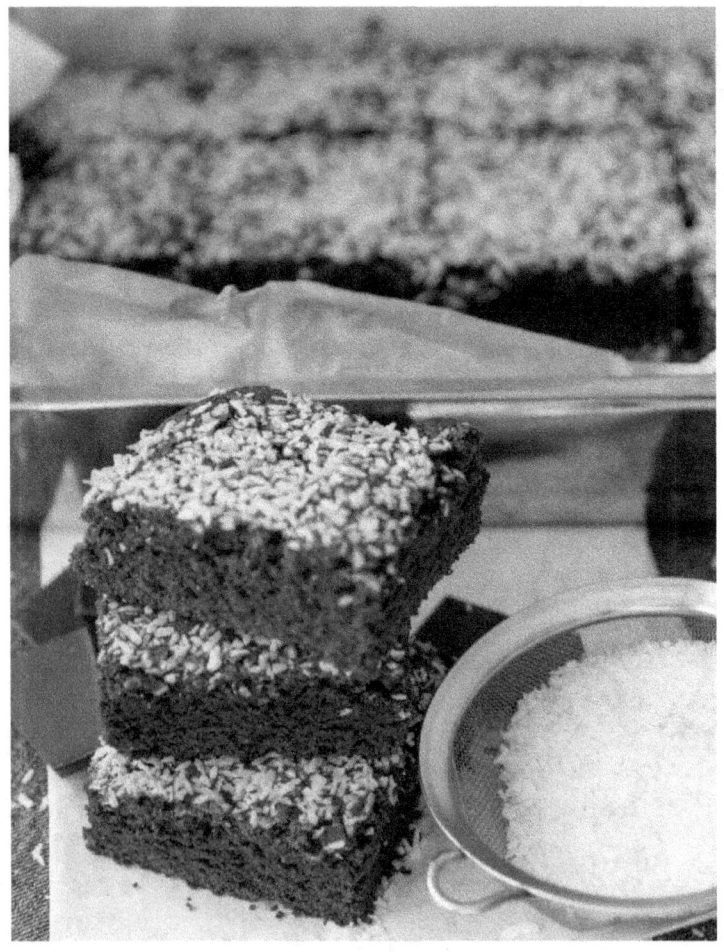

Preparation time: 5 minutes

cooking time: 35 minutes

servings: 12 brownies

Ingredients

- 1 cup whole-grain flour
- 1 teaspoon baking powder
- 1/2 cup unsweetened cocoa powder
- 1 cup light brown sugar
- 1/2 cup canola oil
- 1/2 teaspoon salt
- ¾ cup unsweetened coconut milk
- 1 teaspoon pure vanilla extract
- 1 teaspoon coconut extract
- 1/2 cup vegan semisweet chocolate chips
- 1/2 cup sweetened shredded coconut

Directions

1. Preheat the oven to 350 °F. Grease an 8-inch square baking pan and set it aside. In a large bowl, combine the flour, cocoa, baking powder, and salt. Set aside.
2. In a medium bowl, mix together the sugar and oil until blended. Stir in the coconut milk

3. and the extracts and blend until smooth. Add the wet ingredients to the dry ingredients, stirring to blend. Fold in the chocolate chips and coconut.
4. Scrape the batter into the prepared baking pan and bake until the center is set and a toothpick inserted in the center comes out clean, 35 to 40 minutes. Let the brownies cool 30 minutes before serving. Store in an airtight container.

Avocado and Rhubarb Salad

Preparation time: 10 minutes

Cooking time: 0 minutes

Servings: 4

Ingredients:

- 1 tablespoon stevia
- 1 cup rhubarb, sliced and boiled
- 1 teaspoon vanilla extract
- 2 avocados, peeled, pitted and sliced
- Juice of 1 lime

Directions:

1. In a bowl, combine the rhubarb with the avocado and the other ingredients, toss and serve.

Nutrition:

calories 140, fat 2, fiber 2, carbs 4, protein 4

Coconut Salad

Preparation time: 10 minutes

Cooking time: 0 minutes

Servings: 6

Ingredients:

- 2 cups coconut flesh, unsweetened and shredded
- 1 tablespoon stevia
- ½ cup walnuts, chopped
- 1 cup blackberries
- 1 tablespoon coconut oil, melted

Directions:

1. In a bowl, combine the coconut with the walnuts and the other ingredients, toss and serve.

Nutrition:

calories 250, fat 23.8, fiber 5.8, carbs 8.9, protein 4.5

Brown Betty Bananas Foster.

Preparation Time: 15 Minutes

Servings: 4

Ingredients:

- 6 cups of cubed white bread, a little stale helps
- 4 ripe bananas, peeled and chopped
- ⅓ cup chopped toasted pecans
- ⅓ cup packed light brown sugar or granulated natural sugar
- ⅓ cup pure maple syrup
- ¼ cup unsweetened almond milk
- 2 tablespoons brandy
- ½ teaspoon ground cinnamon
- ¼ teaspoon ground nutmeg
- ¼ teaspoon ground ginger
- ⅛ teaspoon salt

Directions:

1. Lightly oil a baking tray that will fit in the steamer basket of your Cooker.

2. In a bowl combine almond milk, maple syrup, and the spices.
3. Roll the bread cubes in the milk mix.
4. In another bowl mix the bananas, pecans, brandy, and sugar.
5. Layer your two mixes in the tray: half bread, half banana, half bread, half banana.
6. Pour the minimum amount of water into the base of your Cooker and lower the steamer basket.
7. Seal and cook on Steam for 12 minutes.
8. Release the pressure quickly and set to one side to cool a little.

Smoothie Bowl

Preparation time: 45 minutes

Ingredients:

- 6 Oz. berries, fresh or frozen
- 2 medium frozen bananas
- 1 cup jellified yogurt
- ½ cup Almond milk
- 1 tbsp. Chia seeds
- 1 tbsp. Hemp seeds
- 1 tbsp. Coconut flakes
- Raspberry jam or any other, to taste

Directions:

1. In a blender, mix the bananas with half of the berries until it has a puree consistency.
2. Organize your smoothie in a bowl decorating it in rows with the yogurt spot, the puree and fresh berries and with a pinch of seeds and flakes you have.

Lemon Curd Dessert (Sugar Free)

Preparation time: 35 minutes

Ingredients:

- 6 egg yolks
- ½ cup unsalted butter
- ½ cup lemon juice
- 2 tbsp. lemon zest
- Stevia for sweetening

Directions:

1. On low heat melt the butter in a saucepan.
2. Whisk in the stevia or any other sweetener, lemon ingredients until combined, then add the egg yolks and return to the stove again over the low heat.
3. Whisk it until the curd starts thickening.
4. Strain into a small bowl and let cool.
5. Can be stored in a fridge for several weeks.

Strawberries Cream

Preparation time: 10 minutes

Cooking time: 0 minutes

Servings: 2

Ingredients:

- 1 cup strawberries, chopped
- 1 cup coconut cream
- ½ teaspoon vanilla extract
- 1 tablespoon stevia

Directions:

1. In a blender, combine the strawberries with the cream and the other ingredients, pulse well, divide into cups and serve cold.

Nutrition:

calories 182, fat 3.1, fiber 2.3, carbs 3.5, protein 2

Blackberry Pie

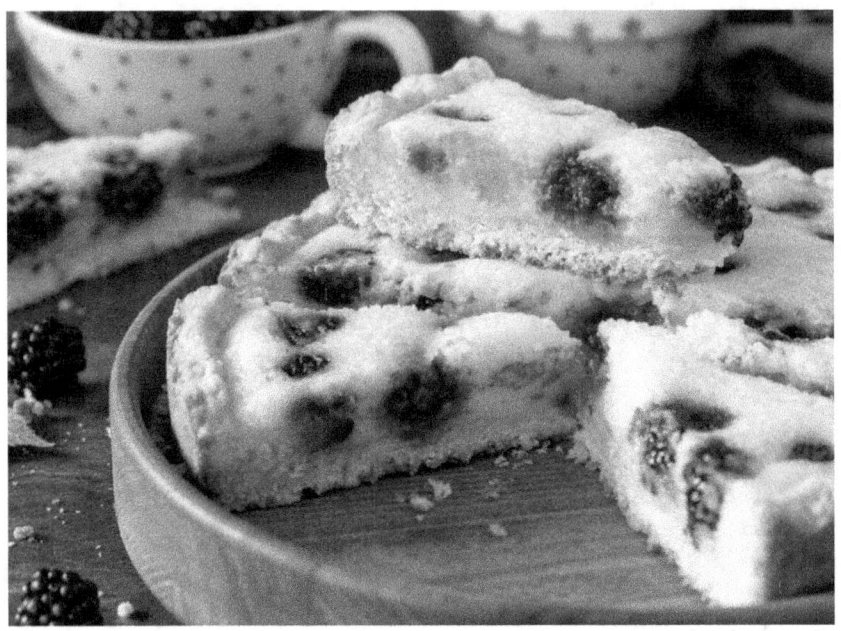

Preparation time: 10 minutes

Cooking time: 35 minutes

Servings: 6

Ingredients:

- ¾ cup stevia
- cups blackberries
- 1 tablespoon lime juice
- ¼ teaspoon baking soda

- 1 cup coconut flour
- ½ cup water
- 3 tablespoons avocado oil
- Cooking spray

Directions:

1. In a bowl, combine the blackberries with the stevia, baking soda and the other ingredients, stir well and transfer to a pie pan.
2. Introduce the pan in the oven at 375 degrees F, bake for 35 minutes, slice and serve warm.

Nutrition:

calories 231, fat 5.5, fiber 24, carbs 42.3, protein 7.2

Lime Cream

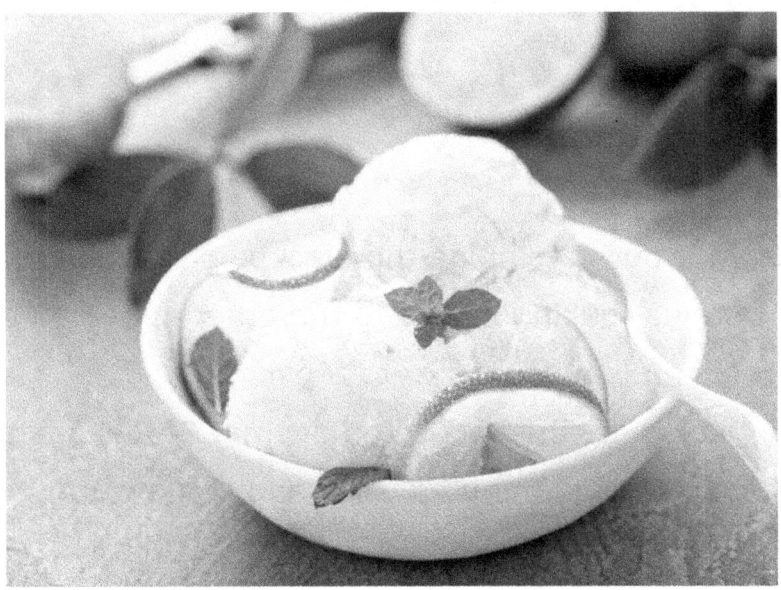

Preparation time: 1 hour

Cooking time: 0 minutes

Servings: 6

Ingredients:

- 2 tablespoons flaxseed mixed with 3 tablespoons water
- 1 cup stevia

- Juice of 1 lime
- 5 tablespoons avocado oil
- 1 cup coconut cream
- Zest of 1 lime, grated

Directions:

1. In a blender, combine the flaxseed mix with the stevia, the oil and the other ingredients, pulse well, divide into cups and keep in the fridge for 1 hour before serving.

Nutrition:

calories 200, fat 8.5, fiber 4.5, carbs 8.6, protein 4.5

Quick And Easy Ranch Dip

Preparation time: 10 minutes plus 4hrs chill time

Cooking time: 0 minutes

Servings: 12

Ingredients:

- 1 cup heavy (whipping) cream
- 1 tablespoon white distilled vinegar
- ¾ cup plain full-fat Greek yogurt
- 1 teaspoon dried dill
- 1 teaspoon freshly squeezed lemon juice
- 2 teaspoons dried parsley
- 1 teaspoon dried chives
- ½ teaspoon garlic powder
- ½ teaspoon onion powder
- ½ teaspoon salt
- ¼ teaspoon freshly ground black pepper

Directions:

1. In a quart-size canning jar, combine the heavy cream and vinegar. Set aside for 5 minutes.

2. Add the Greek yogurt and lemon juice and stir (or shake the jar) well.
3. Add the parsley, dill, chives, garlic powder, onion powder, salt, and pepper, and stir until thoroughly mixed.
4. Put the lid on the jar and place in the refrigerator for 4 hours or overnight for the flavors to combine.

Nutritions:

Calories 79, fat 7g, protein 2g, carbs: 2g; fiber 0g, sugar 2g, sodium 109mg

Roasted Cashews

Preparation Time: 5 minutes

Cooking Time: 3 hours

Servings: 4

Ingredients:

- 1 cup cashews
- 1 cup water
- 2 tablespoons cinnamon

Directions:

1. Add water and cashews to a bowl and soak overnight. Drain the cashews and place on a paper towel to dry. Preheat oven to 200° Fahrenheit. Place the soaked cashews on a baking tray. Sprinkle cashews with cinnamon. Roast in preheated oven for 3 hours. Allow cooling time and then serve and enjoy!

Nutritions:

Calories: 205 Sugar: 1.8 g Fat: 15.9 g Carbohydrates: 13.9 g Cholesterol: 0 mg Protein: 5.4 g

Brownies

Preparation Time: 10 minutes

Cooking time: 15 minutes

Servings: 16

Ingredients:

- 1 cup almond milk yogurt
- ½ teaspoon baking powder
- 2 cups almond flour
- 4 tablespoon cocoa powder
- 1 teaspoon vanilla extract
- ½ cup Erythritol
- ¾ teaspoon salt
- 1 tablespoon flax meal

Directions:

1. Preheat the oven to 355 °F.
2. In the mixing bowl, combine together all the dry ingredients.
3. Then add almond milk yogurt and stir the mixture until you get the batter.

4. Line the tray with the baking paper and transfer batter on it.
5. Flatten brownie batter with the help of a spatula.
6. Place the brownie in the preheated oven and cook for 15 minutes.
7. Then remove the tray with a brownie from the oven.
8. Cut the brownie into 16 serving bars.
9. Transfer the brownie bars in the fridge for 6 hours.

Nutritions:

Calories 100, fat 7.8, fiber 2, carbs 10, protein 3.7

Rich Jackfruit Dish

Preparation time: 10 minutes

Cooking time: 6 hours

Servings: 4

Ingredients:

- ½ cup tamari
- 40 ounces canned young jackfruit, drained
- ¼ cup coconut aminos
- ½ cup agave nectar
- 1 cup mirin
- 8 garlic cloves, minced
- 2 tablespoons ginger, grated
- 1 yellow onion, chopped
- 4 tablespoons sesame oil
- 1 green pear, cored and chopped
- ½ cup water

Directions:

1. In your slow cooker, mix tamari with jackfruit, aminos, mirin, agave nectar, garlic, ginger, onion, sesame oil, water and pear, stir, cover

and cook on Low for 6 hours.
2. Divide into bowls and serve.
3. Enjoy!

Nutritions:

Calories 160, fat 4, fiber 1, carbs 20, protein 4

Avocado Pudding

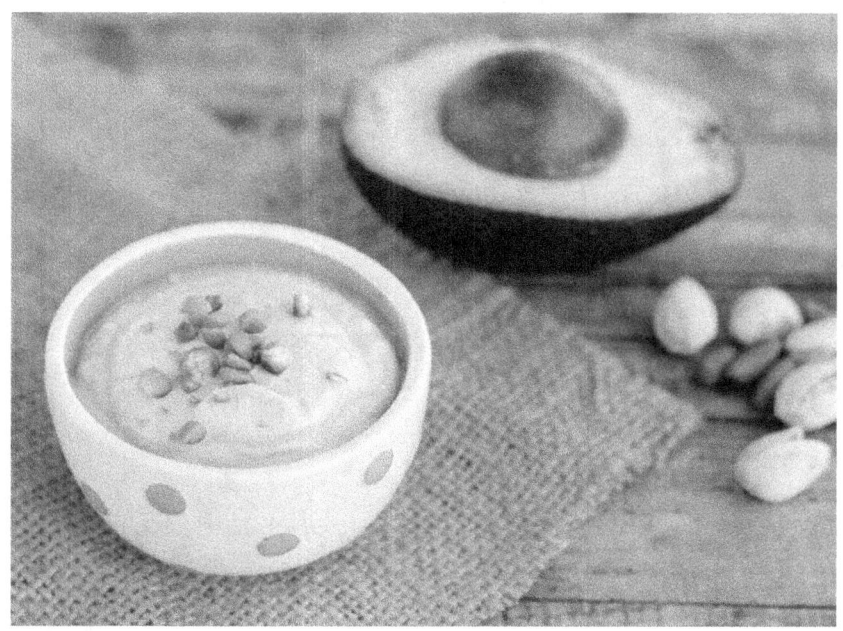

Preparation Time: 10 minutes

Cooking Time: 0 minute

Servings: 8

Ingredients:

- 2 ripe avocados, peeled, pitted and cut into pieces
- 1 tbsp fresh lime juice

- 80 drops of liquid stevia
- 14 oz can coconut milk
- 2 tsp vanilla extract

Directions:

1. Add all ingredients into the blender and blend until smooth.
2. Serve and enjoy.

Nutritions:

Calories 317, Fat 30.1g. Carbohydrates 9.3g, Sugar 0.4g, Protein 3.4g, Cholesterol 0mg

Avocado and Almond Sweet Cream

Preparation time: 20 minutes

Cooking time: 0 minutes

Servings: 6

Ingredients:

- 2 avocados, peeled, pitted and mashed
- 1 cup coconut cream
- 2 tablespoons stevia
- ¾ cup stevia
- 1 teaspoon almond extract
- ¾ cup almonds, ground

Directions:

1. In a blender, combine the avocados with the cream and the other ingredients, pulse well, divide into cups and keep in the fridge for at least 20 minutes before serving.

Nutrition:

Calories 106, fat 3.4, fiber 0, carbs 2.4, protein 4

NOTE

www.ingramcontent.com/pod-product-compliance
Lightning Source LLC
Chambersburg PA
CBHW070934080526
44589CB00013B/1505